Understanding Cancer

A Comprehensive Guide to Diagnosis, Treatment, and Prevention

By

JOEL K. JOHN

TABLE OF CONTENT

Chapter 1: Introduction to Cancer

Understanding Cancer: Definition and Basic Concepts

Cancer, also known as malignant neoplasm, is a complex and diverse group of diseases characterized by uncontrolled cell growth and proliferation. In this chapter, we will explore the fundamental aspects of cancer, its definition, and the basic concepts that underlie its development and progression.

What Is Cancer?

Cancer can be defined as a disease that arises when cells in a specific part of the body undergo uncontrollable growth, fail to follow the normal cell cycle, and form a mass of abnormal tissue called a tumor.

These tumor cells have the ability to invade surrounding tissues and, in some cases, spread to distant parts of the body through a process known as metastasis.

Cancer can occur in virtually any tissue or organ in the body and can manifest as a broad range of diseases, each with its unique characteristics and treatment challenges. The most common types of cancer include breast cancer, lung cancer, prostate cancer, colorectal cancer, and skin cancer, among others.

1.2 Basic Concepts of Cancer Development

Several key concepts are essential to understanding how cancer develops and progresses:

1.2.1 **Genetic Mutations**: At the core of cancer development are genetic mutations, which are alterations in the DNA sequence of genes. Mutations can lead to abnormal cell behavior, disrupt the regulation of the cell cycle, and promote uncontrolled cell growth.

1.2.2 Oncogenes and Tumor Suppressors

Oncogenes are genes that have the potential to cause cancer when mutated or overexpressed. They promote cell proliferation and survival. In contrast, tumor suppressor genes normally inhibit cell growth and division but become ineffective when mutated, allowing cancer to develop.

1.2.3 Carcinogenesis

Carcinogenesis is the process by which normal cells transform into cancer cells. This transformation often involves multiple genetic mutations and epigenetic changes that gradually confer the hallmarks of cancer.

1.2.4 Tumor Microenvironment

The tumor microenvironment includes the cells, blood vessels, and connective tissue surrounding a tumor. It plays a crucial role in tumor growth, invasion, and metastasis, as well as interactions with the immune system.

1.3 Risk Factors for Cancer

Cancer development is influenced by a combination of genetic and environmental factors. Some of the common risk factors include:

1.3.1 **Age**: Cancer incidence increases with age, as accumulated genetic mutations over time raise the risk of developing cancer.

1.3.2 **Lifestyle Factors**: Certain lifestyle choices, such as tobacco and alcohol use, poor diet, lack of physical activity, and exposure to environmental carcinogens, can increase the risk of cancer.

1.3.3 **Genetic Predisposition**: Inherited genetic mutations can significantly increase the likelihood of developing certain types of cancer.

1.3.4 **Chronic Inflammation**: Long-term inflammation in certain tissues can create a favorable environment for cancer development.

Understanding cancer is crucial in the fight against this complex disease. Cancer is a result of genetic mutations and dysregulation of cell growth, leading to the formation of tumors that can invade nearby tissues and spread throughout the body. Recognizing the basic concepts of cancer development and the risk factors involved will pave the way for effective prevention, early detection, and innovative treatment strategies to combat cancer and improve patient outcomes.

The History of Cancer Research

The history of cancer research is a remarkable journey that spans centuries of human curiosity, perseverance, and scientific advancement. From ancient times to the modern era, humanity has endeavored to unravel the mysteries of cancer, understand its causes, and develop effective treatments. This chapter delves into the key milestones and breakthroughs that have shaped our understanding of cancer and paved the way for improved cancer care.

Ancient Observations and Early Beliefs
The roots of cancer research can be traced back to ancient civilizations such as Egypt, Greece, and Rome. Ancient physicians, including Hippocrates, described various tumors and attempted to categorize them based on their appearance and behavior. However, in the absence of modern scientific tools, the understanding of cancer remained limited, and early beliefs

often attributed cancer to imbalances in bodily fluids or divine punishment.

The Emergence of Cancer Surgery

One of the earliest known attempts to treat cancer dates back to ancient Egypt, where records indicate attempts at removing tumors through surgical means. In ancient times, surgery was primarily aimed at relieving symptoms caused by tumors rather than curing the disease. It wasn't until the Middle Ages that more systematic approaches to tumor removal were developed, albeit with limited success.

Advancements in Anatomical Understanding

The Renaissance period brought significant advancements in the understanding of human anatomy, thanks to pioneers like Andreas Vesalius. This improved knowledge of human anatomy laid the groundwork for more accurate descriptions and classifications of tumors, enhancing the accuracy of diagnosis and enabling better-targeted treatments.

The Rise of Experimental Science

The scientific revolution of the 17th century ushered in a new era of experimental science. However, cancer research progress remained slow due to the lack of precise tools to study cellular and molecular mechanisms. The work of Giovanni Morgagni, considered the father of anatomical pathology, marked a turning point as he correlated postmortem findings with clinical symptoms.

Cellular Discoveries and Pathology

The 19th century witnessed significant developments in cellular biology, which greatly influenced cancer research. Rudolf Virchow proposed the concept of "cellular pathology" and identified abnormal cell division as a key characteristic of cancer. His work laid the foundation for understanding cancer as a disease of cellular proliferation.

Discoveries in Radiation and Chemotherapy

The 20th century brought significant progress in cancer research. Wilhelm Conrad Roentgen's discovery of X-rays in 1895 opened the door to the use of radiation therapy for cancer treatment. The development of chemotherapeutic agents, such as nitrogen mustard during World War II, marked a critical step forward in systemic cancer treatment.

Unraveling the Genetic Basis of Cancer

Advances in molecular biology and genetics in the latter half of the 20th century revolutionized cancer research. The discovery of oncogenes and tumor suppressor genes, such as the retinoblastoma (Rb) gene and the p53 gene, provided profound insights into the genetic basis of cancer development.

Targeted Therapies and Immunotherapy

Recent decades have seen an explosion of research into targeted therapies and immunotherapy. The identification of specific molecular targets and the development of monoclonal antibodies, tyrosine kinase inhibitors, and immune checkpoint inhibitors have transformed cancer treatment, leading to improved outcomes for many patients.

Precision Medicine and Personalized Therapy

The advent of advanced genomic technologies has enabled the emergence of precision medicine. Molecular profiling of tumors allows oncologists to tailor treatment plans to individual patients based on the unique genetic characteristics of their cancer.

The history of cancer research is a testament to the tireless efforts of countless researchers and medical professionals who have dedicated their lives to understanding and combating this formidable disease. From ancient observations to modern molecular insights, each discovery has contributed to the progress in cancer care and continues to drive us forward in the pursuit of better prevention, diagnosis, and treatment options for cancer patients.

Types of Cancer: An Overview

Cancer is not a single disease but rather a collection of diverse and complex conditions that can affect virtually any part of the body. The vast array of cancer types is a result of the different tissues and organs in which abnormal cell growth can occur. In this chapter, we will provide an overview of some of the most common and significant types of cancer, highlighting their key characteristics and potential risk factors.

Breast Cancer:
Breast cancer is one of the most prevalent cancers among women worldwide. It originates in the breast tissue, commonly in the ducts or lobules. Risk factors for breast cancer include age, family history, hormonal factors, and lifestyle choices. Early detection through regular breast self-examinations, mammograms, and clinical screenings is crucial for improving treatment outcomes.

Lung Cancer:
Lung cancer is a type of cancer that develops in the lungs, typically in the cells lining the air passages. It is strongly associated with tobacco smoking, but non-smokers can also develop lung cancer due to exposure to environmental carcinogens. Early symptoms may be subtle, leading to late-stage diagnoses. Lung cancer is categorized into two main types: non-small cell lung cancer (NSCLC) and small cell lung cancer (SCLC).

Colorectal Cancer:
Colorectal cancer affects the colon or rectum and usually starts as polyps, which are abnormal growths in the inner lining of these organs. If left untreated, some polyps can turn into cancer over time. Regular screening through colonoscopies can help detect and remove polyps before they become cancerous. Lifestyle factors, such as a high-fat diet and sedentary lifestyle, can increase the risk of colorectal cancer.

Prostate Cancer:
Prostate cancer is a cancer that affects the prostate gland, which is part of the male reproductive system. It is the most common cancer in men and is often slow-growing. Risk factors include age, family history, and certain genetic mutations. Prostate-specific antigen (PSA) testing and digital rectal examination are used for early detection and monitoring.

Skin Cancer:
Skin cancer develops in the cells of the skin and is primarily caused by exposure to ultraviolet (UV) radiation from the sun or artificial sources like tanning beds. The main types of skin cancer are basal cell carcinoma, squamous cell carcinoma, and melanoma. Melanoma is the most dangerous form of skin cancer due to its potential to spread to other parts of the body.

Leukemia:
Leukemia is a cancer of the blood and bone marrow, characterized by the rapid production of abnormal white blood cells. These abnormal cells interfere with the production of healthy blood cells and weaken the immune system. Leukemia can be classified into several types, including acute lymphoblastic leukemia (ALL), acute myeloid leukemia (AML), chronic lymphocytic leukemia (CLL), and chronic myeloid leukemia (CML).

Lymphoma:
Lymphoma is a cancer that originates in the lymphatic system, a part of the immune system. There are two main types of lymphoma: Hodgkin lymphoma and non-Hodgkin lymphoma. Both types involve the abnormal growth of lymphocytes, which are a type of white blood cell.

Ovarian Cancer:
Ovarian cancer arises in the ovaries, the female reproductive organs that produce eggs. It is often challenging to detect in its early stages, leading to a higher likelihood of being diagnosed at an advanced stage. Risk factors for ovarian cancer include family history, genetic mutations, and hormonal factors.

Cancer encompasses a broad range of diseases affecting different organs and tissues in the body. Early detection and awareness of risk factors are crucial in improving the prognosis for individuals diagnosed with cancer. Continued research and advances in cancer treatment and prevention hold the promise of further enhancing outcomes for patients and reducing the global burden of cancer.

Chapter 2: Causes and Risk Factors

Genetic Factors: Oncogenes and Tumor Suppressors

Genetic factors play a significant role in the development of cancer. Mutations or alterations in specific genes can lead to the dysregulation of cell growth and division, contributing to the formation and progression of tumors. Two critical types of genes involved in cancer development are oncogenes and tumor suppressor genes. In this chapter, we will explore the roles of oncogenes and tumor suppressors and how their dysregulation can lead to the initiation and promotion of cancer.

Oncogenes:
Oncogenes are a class of genes that have the potential to transform normal cells into cancerous cells when mutated or activated.

Normally, these genes play crucial roles in regulating cell growth, cell division, and cell differentiation. However, when an oncogene undergoes a gain-of-function mutation or other activating alterations, it can drive excessive and uncontrolled cell proliferation, a hallmark of cancer.

Activation of oncogenes can occur through various mechanisms, such as:

Point mutations: Single nucleotide changes in the DNA sequence of the oncogene can lead to its constitutive activation.

Gene amplification: The oncogene is duplicated or amplified, resulting in increased gene expression and protein production.

Chromosomal translocations: A portion of the oncogene is rearranged and fused with a different gene, leading to its activation and the creation of a fusion protein with oncogenic properties.

Examples of well-known oncogenes include:

-HER2 (Human Epidermal Growth Factor Receptor 2) in breast cancer.
-RAS genes (KRAS, NRAS, HRAS) in various cancers, including colorectal cancer.
-BCR-ABL fusion gene in chronic myeloid leukemia (CML).

Tumor Suppressor Genes:
Tumor suppressor genes, as the name suggests, act as "brakes" in the cell cycle and play a critical role in preventing the development of cancer. Their normal function is to inhibit cell growth, promote repair of damaged DNA, and induce apoptosis (cell death) when necessary. Loss or inactivation of tumor suppressor genes removes these inhibitory signals, allowing cells to divide uncontrollably and escape programmed cell death, leading to cancer initiation and progression.

Tumor suppressor genes can be inactivated through various mechanisms, such as:

Loss-of-function mutations: Mutations that disrupt the normal function of the tumor suppressor gene.
Gene deletion: The entire gene or a significant portion of it is lost from the genome.
Epigenetic silencing: Chemical modifications to the DNA or histone proteins result in decreased gene expression without altering the gene sequence.

Examples of well-known tumor suppressor genes include:

TP53 (p53): Often referred to as the "guardian of the genome," mutations in TP53 are found in a wide range of cancers.

RB1 (Retinoblastoma 1): Mutations in RB1 are associated with retinoblastoma and other cancers.

BRCA1 and BRCA2: Mutations in these genes increase the risk of breast and ovarian cancer.

The balance between oncogenes and tumor suppressor genes is crucial for maintaining normal cell growth and preventing cancer. When mutations tip this balance in favor of uncontrolled cell proliferation, cancer can develop. Understanding the role of these genetic factors in cancer has paved the way for targeted therapies that aim to inhibit oncogenes or reactivate tumor suppressors, providing promising approaches to cancer treatment and personalized medicine.

Environmental Carcinogens and Lifestyle Factors

Cancer development is influenced not only by genetic factors but also by environmental and lifestyle factors. Exposure to certain substances in the environment, as well as lifestyle choices, can significantly increase the risk of developing cancer. In this chapter, we will explore the impact of environmental carcinogens and lifestyle factors on cancer risk and how understanding these influences can help in cancer prevention and public health strategies.

Environmental Carcinogens:
Environmental carcinogens are substances present in the environment that have the potential to cause cancer. These carcinogens can be found in various forms, including chemical, physical, and biological agents. Prolonged or repeated exposure to these agents can damage the DNA within cells, leading to genetic

mutations and the initiation of cancer. Some common environmental carcinogens include:

Tobacco Smoke: Cigarette smoking is the leading cause of preventable cancer deaths worldwide. Tobacco smoke contains numerous carcinogens that can affect various organs, including the lungs, throat, mouth, esophagus, and bladder.

Air Pollutants: Certain air pollutants, such as benzene, formaldehyde, and particulate matter, have been linked to an increased risk of lung cancer and other respiratory system cancers.

Occupational Exposures: Some professions involve exposure to carcinogenic substances. For example, asbestos exposure is associated with lung cancer and mesothelioma, a rare cancer affecting the lining of the lungs and other organs.

Ultraviolet (UV) Radiation: Excessive exposure to UV radiation from the sun or artificial sources like tanning beds can lead to skin cancer, including melanoma, basal cell carcinoma, and squamous cell carcinoma.

Ionizing Radiation: High-dose ionizing radiation, such as from medical imaging procedures or radiation therapy, can increase the risk of cancer development.

Lifestyle Factors:
Certain lifestyle choices and habits can also impact cancer risk. Adopting healthy behaviors can help reduce the likelihood of developing cancer. Some lifestyle factors that influence cancer risk include:

Diet: A diet high in processed foods, red meat, and saturated fats may contribute to an increased risk of cancer, particularly colorectal and stomach cancers. On the other hand, a diet rich in fruits, vegetables, whole grains, and lean proteins can have a protective effect.

Physical Inactivity: Lack of regular physical activity is associated with an increased risk of several cancers, including breast, colon, and prostate cancers.

Obesity: Being overweight or obese is linked to an elevated risk of developing various cancers, including breast, endometrial, and kidney cancers.

Alcohol Consumption: Excessive alcohol consumption can increase the risk of developing several types of cancer, including liver, esophageal, and breast cancers.

Tobacco and E-Cigarette Use: Tobacco use, including smoking and smokeless tobacco, is a well-established cause of cancer. Similarly, the long-term health effects of e-cigarette use are still under investigation, but they may also pose cancer risks.

Understanding the impact of environmental carcinogens and lifestyle factors on cancer risk is essential for public health efforts aimed at cancer prevention. By raising awareness of these risk factors and promoting healthier behaviors, we can potentially reduce the incidence of cancer and improve overall population health. Additionally, regulation and mitigation of exposure to environmental carcinogens can play a critical role in preventing cancer in vulnerable populations.

The Role of Chronic Inflammation in Cancer Development

Inflammation is a natural response of the immune system to injury, infection, or harmful stimuli. It is a vital process that helps the body eliminate pathogens, repair damaged tissues, and restore normal function. However, when inflammation becomes chronic and persists over an extended period, it can contribute to various diseases, including cancer. In this chapter, we will explore the role of chronic inflammation in cancer development and how understanding this relationship can lead to better strategies for cancer prevention and treatment.

Acute vs. Chronic Inflammation: Acute inflammation is a short-term and localized response to tissue injury or infection. It involves the activation of immune cells, release of inflammatory mediators (e.g., cytokines and chemokines), and increased blood flow to the affected area, leading to redness, heat, swelling, and pain.

On the other hand, chronic inflammation is a sustained and prolonged inflammatory response that can last for weeks, months, or even years. Unlike acute inflammation, chronic inflammation involves the infiltration of immune cells into the affected tissues, causing persistent tissue damage and remodeling.

Inflammatory Response and Cancer Development:

Chronic inflammation creates an environment conducive to cancer development and progression through several mechanisms:

DNA Damage: Inflammatory mediators and reactive oxygen species released during chronic inflammation can cause DNA damage in the affected cells. DNA damage, if not adequately repaired, can lead to the accumulation of genetic mutations that promote cancer initiation.

Cell Proliferation: Inflammatory signals can stimulate cell proliferation to promote tissue repair. However, when uncontrolled, this cell proliferation can also contribute to the growth of cancer cells.

Angiogenesis: Chronic inflammation can induce the formation of new blood vessels (angiogenesis) to supply nutrients and oxygen to the inflamed tissues. This process can also support the growth and survival of cancer cells by providing them with the necessary resources.

Immune Suppression: Prolonged inflammation can lead to immune suppression, compromising the immune system's ability to recognize and eliminate cancer cells effectively.

Examples of Chronic Inflammatory Conditions and Associated Cancers: Several chronic inflammatory conditions are associated with an increased risk of cancer:

Chronic Hepatitis: Chronic hepatitis B and C infections are linked to an elevated risk of liver cancer (hepatocellular carcinoma).

Inflammatory Bowel Disease (IBD): Ulcerative colitis and Crohn's disease, both forms of IBD, are associated with an increased risk of colorectal cancer.

Chronic Gastritis: Long-term inflammation of the stomach lining due to Helicobacter pylori infection is a risk factor for gastric (stomach) cancer.

Chronic Pancreatitis: Prolonged inflammation of the pancreas is associated with an increased risk of pancreatic cancer.

Chronic Lung Diseases: Chronic inflammation caused by conditions such as chronic obstructive pulmonary disease (COPD) and pulmonary fibrosis may elevate the risk of lung cancer.

Targeting Chronic Inflammation for Cancer Prevention and Treatment: Given the link between chronic inflammation and cancer development, researchers are exploring strategies to target inflammation as a means of cancer prevention and treatment. Anti-inflammatory drugs, such as nonsteroidal anti-inflammatory drugs (NSAIDs), have shown potential in reducing cancer risk and slowing cancer progression in some cases. Additionally, lifestyle modifications, such as quitting smoking and adopting a healthy diet, can help reduce chronic inflammation and lower cancer risk.

Chronic inflammation plays a critical role in cancer development by promoting DNA damage, cell proliferation, angiogenesis, and immune suppression. Understanding the complex relationship between chronic inflammation and cancer is essential for developing effective strategies for cancer prevention and treatment.

By addressing the underlying causes of chronic inflammation and intervening at the molecular level, we can potentially reduce cancer incidence and improve patient outcomes.

Chapter 3: Pathophysiology of Cancer

Cell Cycle and Regulation

The cell cycle is a highly regulated and orchestrated process that governs the growth, division, and duplication of cells. It plays a fundamental role in tissue growth, repair, and maintenance, as well as in the development and progression of various diseases, including cancer. In this chapter, we will explore the cell cycle, its different phases, and the intricate regulatory mechanisms that ensure proper cell division and function.

The Cell Cycle:
The cell cycle is a series of events that occur in a eukaryotic cell leading to its division into two daughter cells. It consists of four distinct phases:

1.1 **G1 Phase (Gap 1 Phase)**: The G1 phase is the first gap phase, where the cell grows and prepares for DNA synthesis (replication). During this phase, the cell synthesizes proteins, RNA, and other components necessary for DNA replication and cell division.

1.2 **S Phase (Synthesis Phase)**: In the S phase, DNA replication occurs, resulting in the duplication of the cell's genetic material. Each chromosome is replicated, forming two sister chromatids held together by a centromere.

1.3 **G2 Phase (Gap 2 Phase)**: The G2 phase is the second gap phase, during which the cell continues to grow and prepares for cell division. It synthesizes additional proteins and organelles required for mitosis (nuclear division) and cytokinesis (cell division).

1.4 **M Phase (Mitotic Phase)**: The M phase is the phase of active cell division, comprising two essential processes:

mitosis and cytokinesis. Mitosis is the division of the cell nucleus, while cytokinesis is the division of the cytoplasm to produce two separate daughter cells.

Cell Cycle Regulation:
The cell cycle is precisely regulated by a complex network of molecular checkpoints and signaling pathways. The key regulators of the cell cycle are a group of proteins called cyclins and cyclin-dependent kinases (CDKs). These proteins work together to control the progression of the cell cycle from one phase to the next.

The cyclin-CDK complexes act as molecular switches, activating various proteins that drive the cell cycle forward or arresting the cycle if errors or DNA damage are detected. Additionally, there are tumor suppressor proteins, such as p53 and RB (Retinoblastoma), which play crucial roles in halting the cell cycle in response to DNA damage or other abnormalities.

Checkpoints in the Cell Cycle:
The cell cycle is subject to several checkpoints, which act as surveillance mechanisms to ensure the integrity and accuracy of cell division. The main checkpoints are:

3.1 **G1 Checkpoint**: This checkpoint occurs at the end of the G1 phase. It assesses whether the cell's environment is favorable for cell division and whether the cell's DNA is intact and ready for replication. If conditions are not suitable, the cell can enter a non-dividing state called G0 phase or undergo apoptosis (programmed cell death).

3.2 **G2 Checkpoint**: This checkpoint occurs at the end of the G2 phase. It verifies that DNA replication was successful and that the cell is ready for mitosis. If DNA damage is detected, the cell cycle is arrested to allow time for repair.

3.3 **Spindle Checkpoint**: This checkpoint occurs during mitosis and ensures that all chromosomes are properly attached to the mitotic spindle before the cell proceeds to complete cell division. If any errors are detected, the process is halted to prevent unequal distribution of genetic material to the daughter cells.

Dysregulation of the Cell Cycle and Cancer:

Dysregulation of the cell cycle is a hallmark of cancer. Cancer cells often acquire mutations in key cell cycle regulatory genes, leading to uncontrolled cell proliferation, genomic instability, and resistance to cell death. Mutations in oncogenes or loss of tumor suppressor function can disrupt the delicate balance of cell cycle control, promoting the formation and growth of cancerous tumors.

Understanding the intricacies of cell cycle regulation is vital for cancer research and the development of targeted therapies. By targeting specific cell cycle checkpoints or key regulatory molecules, researchers aim to selectively inhibit the growth of cancer cells while sparing normal cells, thereby providing more effective and less toxic treatments for cancer patients.

Oncogenesis: The Process of Tumorigenesis

Oncogenesis, also known as tumorigenesis or carcinogenesis, is the process by which normal cells transform into cancer cells. It is a complex and multistep process involving genetic and epigenetic changes that disrupt the normal regulation of cell growth, leading to uncontrolled proliferation and the formation of tumors. In this chapter, we will explore the key stages and factors involved in oncogenesis and the factors that contribute to the development of cancer.

Initiation:

The first stage of oncogenesis is initiation, which involves the initial genetic damage or mutation in a normal cell. This mutation can be caused by various factors, such as exposure to carcinogens (chemical, physical, or biological agents that can induce cancer), radiation, or spontaneous errors during DNA replication. The mutated cell retains the ability to divide and pass on its genetic alterations to daughter cells.

Promotion:
Following initiation, the initiated cell may enter the promotion stage. During this stage, further genetic alterations and epigenetic changes occur in the initiated cell, resulting in the expansion and clonal expansion of the mutated cells. Promotion is often a reversible process, and if the promoting agent is removed, the cells may revert to a normal phenotype.

Progression:
Progression is the final stage of tumorigenesis, characterized by the development of a fully malignant phenotype. In this stage, the transformed cells acquire additional genetic alterations that enhance their ability to proliferate, invade surrounding tissues, and metastasize to distant sites. These changes lead to the formation of a clinically detectable tumor and its spread to other parts of the body.

Factors Contributing to Oncogenesis:

Several factors contribute to the development of oncogenesis:

Genetic Mutations: Mutations in critical genes involved in cell cycle regulation, DNA repair, and apoptosis can disrupt normal cellular processes, leading to uncontrolled cell growth and survival.

Oncogenes and Tumor Suppressors: Activation of oncogenes and inactivation of tumor suppressor genes play a central role in driving oncogenesis. Oncogenes promote cell proliferation, while tumor suppressors inhibit it. Dysregulation of these genes can lead to uncontrolled cell division.

Chronic Inflammation: Prolonged inflammation creates an environment conducive to oncogenesis. Inflammatory cells release reactive oxygen species and inflammatory mediators that can cause

DNA damage and promote cell proliferation.

Environmental Carcinogens: Exposure to environmental carcinogens, such as tobacco smoke, ultraviolet radiation, and certain chemicals, can induce genetic mutations and contribute to the initiation of oncogenesis.

Viral Infections: Some viruses, such as human papillomavirus (HPV), hepatitis B virus (HBV), and human immunodeficiency virus (HIV), can integrate their DNA into host cells and disrupt normal cellular functions, leading to cancer development.

Epigenetic Changes: Epigenetic modifications, such as DNA methylation and histone modifications, can alter gene expression patterns without changing the underlying DNA sequence. Epigenetic changes can silence tumor suppressor genes or activate oncogenes, contributing to oncogenesis.

Understanding the process of tumorigenesis is crucial for cancer research and the development of targeted therapies. By identifying the key genetic and molecular events driving oncogenesis, researchers can design therapies that specifically target these processes, providing more effective and personalized treatments for cancer patients. Additionally, early detection and intervention during the stages of initiation and promotion can potentially prevent the progression of oncogenesis and improve cancer outcomes.

Angiogenesis and Metastasis

Angiogenesis and metastasis are two critical processes in the progression and spread of cancer. Both phenomena play pivotal roles in the development of advanced and aggressive forms of cancer. In this chapter, we will explore the significance of angiogenesis and metastasis in cancer biology and their implications for cancer treatment and patient prognosis.

Angiogenesis:
Angiogenesis is the process of new blood vessel formation from pre-existing vessels. In normal physiological conditions, angiogenesis occurs during tissue growth, wound healing, and the female reproductive cycle. However, in the context of cancer, angiogenesis plays a crucial role in tumor growth and progression.

Cancer cells release pro-angiogenic factors, such as vascular endothelial growth factor (VEGF) and platelet-derived growth factor (PDGF), which stimulate nearby blood vessels to grow and sprout new capillaries toward the tumor mass. These new blood vessels supply the growing tumor with oxygen and nutrients, facilitating its expansion and enabling it to survive and thrive in the surrounding tissue.

Inhibiting angiogenesis has become a significant therapeutic approach in cancer treatment. Anti-angiogenic drugs aim to block the action of pro-angiogenic factors or target the blood vessels themselves, effectively starving the tumor of its blood supply and impeding its growth.

Metastasis:
Metastasis is the process by which cancer cells spread from the primary tumor site to other parts of the body, forming secondary tumors or metastases. Metastasis is a complex and multistep process involving several stages:

Local Invasion: Cancer cells at the primary tumor site acquire the ability to invade nearby tissues, breaking through the basement membrane and surrounding barriers.

Intravasation: Invading cancer cells enter nearby blood or lymphatic vessels, allowing them to travel through the circulation.

Circulation: Cancer cells circulate through the bloodstream or lymphatic system, surviving the harsh conditions and immune surveillance during transit.

Extravasation: Cancer cells exit the blood or lymphatic vessels at distant sites, often in organs or tissues that are more susceptible to colonization.

Colonization: Once at a distant site, cancer cells adapt to the new microenvironment, proliferate, and form secondary tumors.

Metastasis is a major challenge in cancer treatment, as it is responsible for most cancer-related deaths. Detecting and treating metastatic tumors can be difficult due to their locations and the potential development of drug resistance.

Targeting Angiogenesis and Metastasis in Cancer Treatment:
Understanding the importance of angiogenesis and metastasis in cancer has led to the development of targeted therapies to address these processes.

Anti-Angiogenic Therapies: Drugs that inhibit angiogenesis, such as bevacizumab and tyrosine kinase inhibitors, have shown promise in slowing tumor growth and improving outcomes in certain cancers.

Metastasis-Inhibiting Therapies: Researchers are actively exploring ways to block specific steps in the metastatic cascade to prevent cancer spread. Novel treatments targeting cancer cell migration, invasion, and colonization are under investigation.

Prognostic Significance:
The presence of angiogenesis and the potential for metastasis are important prognostic indicators in cancer. Tumors with high levels of angiogenesis and a propensity for metastasis are generally associated with more aggressive disease and poorer outcomes.

Angiogenesis and metastasis are critical processes in cancer progression, contributing to tumor growth, spread, and treatment resistance. Targeting these processes has opened new avenues for cancer therapy and holds promise for improving patient outcomes. A comprehensive understanding of angiogenesis and metastasis is essential for designing effective therapeutic strategies and advancing cancer research.

Chapter 4: Cancer Diagnosis and Screening

Early Detection Methods: Screening and Imaging Techniques

Early detection of cancer is crucial for improving treatment outcomes and increasing the chances of successful recovery. Screening and imaging techniques are essential tools in identifying cancer at its early stages when it is more treatable and has a better prognosis. In this chapter, we will explore various early detection methods used in cancer screening and imaging, highlighting their importance in detecting cancer at its earliest and most manageable stage.

Cancer Screening:
Cancer screening involves the systematic examination of individuals who are asymptomatic but at higher risk of developing cancer.

Screening aims to identify early signs of cancer or precancerous changes, enabling early intervention and improved treatment outcomes. Some common cancer screening methods include:

1.1. **Mammography**: Mammograms are X-ray images of the breast tissue used for breast cancer screening. Regular mammography is recommended for women aged 40 and above to detect breast cancer at an early stage.

1.2. **Pap Smear**: The Pap smear is a screening test used to detect precancerous changes in the cells of the cervix. It is a vital tool in cervical cancer prevention and is recommended for women starting at age 21.

1.3. **Colonoscopy**: Colonoscopy is a procedure that allows the visualization of the colon and rectum to detect polyps or abnormal growths that may lead to colorectal cancer. Regular colonoscopy is recommended for adults over 50 years old.

1.4. Prostate-Specific Antigen (PSA) Test: The PSA test measures the level of PSA in the blood, which can be elevated in prostate cancer. It is commonly used for prostate cancer screening in men.

Imaging Techniques:
Imaging techniques are non-invasive procedures used to visualize internal body structures and identify abnormalities, including tumors. Imaging plays a crucial role in cancer diagnosis, staging, and treatment planning. Some common imaging techniques used in cancer diagnosis include:

2.1. X-rays: X-rays are a basic imaging tool used to visualize bone structures and identify abnormalities such as bone metastases. They are commonly used in diagnosing lung cancer and detecting bone-related complications in cancer patients.

2.2. **Computed Tomography (CT)**: CT scans use X-rays to create detailed cross-sectional images of the body. CT scans are valuable for detecting tumors, assessing lymph node involvement, and staging cancers in various organs.

2.3. **Magnetic Resonance Imaging (MRI)**: MRI uses strong magnetic fields and radio waves to create detailed images of soft tissues in the body. It is particularly useful in evaluating the brain, spinal cord, pelvic organs, and breast tissue.

2.4. **Positron Emission Tomography (PET)**: PET scans involve injecting a small amount of radioactive tracer into the body, which is taken up by active cells, including cancer cells. The PET scan detects areas with high metabolic activity, aiding in cancer staging and evaluating treatment response.

Early detection through screening and imaging allows for prompt diagnosis and timely initiation of treatment, potentially improving patient outcomes and increasing the likelihood of successful cancer management. It is essential for individuals to adhere to recommended cancer screening guidelines based on their age, gender, and risk factors, as early detection is a critical factor in the fight against cancer. Additionally, advances in imaging technology continue to improve the accuracy and sensitivity of cancer detection, contributing to better patient care and outcomes.

Biopsy and Histopathology

Biopsy and histopathology are essential procedures used in cancer diagnosis and the evaluation of abnormal tissue growth. They play a crucial role in confirming the presence of cancer, determining the type and grade of the tumor, and guiding treatment decisions. In this chapter, we will explore the significance of biopsies and histopathology in cancer diagnosis and treatment planning.

Biopsy:
A biopsy is a medical procedure in which a small sample of tissue or cells is taken from the suspected area of abnormality for examination under a microscope. Biopsies are performed to diagnose cancer, determine its stage and grade, and identify specific molecular characteristics that can guide targeted therapies. There are different types of biopsies, including:

1.1. **Needle Biopsy**: In a needle biopsy, a thin needle is used to extract a small tissue sample from a tumor or abnormal area. This type of biopsy is often used for tumors located deep within the body or for lesions that are difficult to access.

1.2. **Incisional Biopsy**: An incisional biopsy involves the removal of a portion of the tumor for examination. This type of biopsy is used when the tumor is too large to be completely removed or when it is not safe to remove the entire mass.

1.3. **Excisional Biopsy**: In an excisional biopsy, the entire tumor or abnormal tissue is removed for examination. This type of biopsy is commonly used when the tumor is small and easily accessible.

1.4. **Endoscopic Biopsy**: Endoscopic biopsies are performed using an endoscope, a flexible tube with a camera, to visualize and obtain samples from the inside of organs or body cavities.

Histopathology:
Histopathology is the microscopic examination of tissue samples obtained through biopsy. After the tissue is collected, it is preserved, processed, and stained to highlight cellular structures and identify any abnormalities. A pathologist, a medical doctor specialized in diagnosing diseases through examination of tissues, analyzes the tissue samples under a microscope and issues a pathology report.

Histopathology helps to:

2.1. **Confirm Cancer Diagnosis**:
Histopathological examination confirms whether the tissue sample is cancerous and identifies the type of cancer.

2.2. **Determine Tumor Grade**: Tumor grade refers to how abnormal the cancer cells look under the microscope. It provides information about the aggressiveness of the cancer and its potential to grow and spread.

2.3. **Assess Tumor Margins**:
Histopathology can evaluate the edges or margins of a tumor to determine if cancer cells are present at the surgical margin after tumor removal. Clear margins are important for reducing the risk of cancer recurrence.

2.4. **Identify Molecular Markers**:
Certain molecular markers detected through histopathology can guide targeted therapies, such as hormone receptors in breast cancer or EGFR mutations in lung cancer.

Biopsy and histopathology are crucial steps in the cancer diagnostic process. The information obtained from these procedures is essential for creating an accurate treatment plan tailored to the individual patient's cancer type and characteristics.

The combination of imaging studies, biopsies, and histopathological analysis ensures that cancer patients receive the most appropriate and effective treatment, improving their chances of successful outcomes.

Biomarkers are biological molecules or substances that can be measured in the body and indicate normal or abnormal processes, conditions, or disease states. In cancer diagnosis, biomarkers play a critical role in identifying the presence of cancer, determining its specific type, and guiding treatment decisions. They provide valuable information about the molecular characteristics of a tumor and can aid in predicting prognosis and treatment response. In this chapter, we will explore the significance of biomarkers in cancer diagnosis and their potential applications in personalized medicine.

Types of Biomarkers Used in Cancer Diagnosis:

Genetic Biomarkers: These biomarkers involve the analysis of genetic alterations in cancer cells, such as mutations, amplifications, or translocations. Genetic biomarkers can indicate the presence of specific mutations associated with certain cancer types, helping to identify the origin of the tumor and guide targeted therapies.

Protein Biomarkers: Protein biomarkers involve the measurement of specific proteins that are overexpressed or underexpressed in cancer cells. Some protein biomarkers are associated with particular cancer types and can be used for early detection, diagnosis, and monitoring of treatment response.

Epigenetic Biomarkers: Epigenetic biomarkers involve changes in the regulation of gene expression without alterations in the DNA sequence. DNA methylation and histone modifications are examples of epigenetic changes that can be detected in cancer cells and used as biomarkers.

Circulating Tumor Markers: Circulating tumor markers are biomolecules that can be measured in the blood and indicate the presence of cancer or the progression of the disease. Examples include prostate-specific antigen (PSA) for prostate cancer and carcinoembryonic antigen (CEA) for colorectal cancer.

Applications of Biomarkers in Cancer Diagnosis:

Early Detection: Biomarkers can be used in cancer screening to identify cancer at its earliest stages, before symptoms are apparent. Early detection allows for more effective treatment and improved patient outcomes.

Cancer Subtyping: Biomarkers can help differentiate between different subtypes of cancer based on their molecular characteristics. This information is essential for tailoring treatment strategies to each patient's specific cancer type.

Prognostication: Certain biomarkers are associated with the aggressiveness of cancer and can be used to predict prognosis. This information helps in estimating the likelihood of disease progression and survival.

Treatment Selection: Biomarkers can guide treatment decisions by indicating the potential efficacy of certain therapies. For example, the presence of specific genetic mutations can determine whether a patient will respond to targeted therapies.

Monitoring Treatment Response: Biomarkers can be used to monitor how well a patient is responding to treatment. Changes in biomarker levels over time can indicate the effectiveness of the therapy and the need for adjustments in the treatment plan.

Personalized Medicine and Biomarkers:

Biomarkers are at the core of personalized medicine, an approach that tailors medical treatment to an individual's unique characteristics, including their genetic makeup and molecular profile. By using biomarkers to guide treatment decisions,

physicians can offer patients more targeted
and effective therapies, reducing the risk
of side effects and improving treatment
outcomes.

Biomarkers are valuable tools in cancer
diagnosis, providing crucial information
about the molecular characteristics of
tumors. They help in early detection,
cancer subtyping, prognostication,
treatment selection, and monitoring
treatment response. As research continues
to advance, biomarkers will play an
increasingly significant role in the field of
oncology, leading to more precise and
personalized cancer care.

Chapter 5: Cancer Staging and Grading

TNM Staging System

The TNM staging system is a standardized method used to describe the extent and spread of cancer within a patient's body. It is one of the most widely used and recognized staging systems in oncology and provides valuable information for treatment planning, prognosis prediction, and research purposes. The TNM system classifies tumors based on three key parameters: T, N, and M, representing the primary tumor, regional lymph nodes, and distant metastasis, respectively. In this chapter, we will explore the significance of the TNM staging system and its application in cancer staging.

T: Primary Tumor

The T category describes the size and extent of the primary tumor at its original location. It provides information about the tumor's invasion into surrounding tissues and organs. The T category is usually expressed using increasing numbers or letters (e.g., T0, Tis, T1, T2, etc.) to represent different stages of tumor growth.

T0: No evidence of the primary tumor.
Tis: Carcinoma in situ - Cancer cells are present only in the layer of cells where they first formed and have not invaded deeper tissues.
T1, T2, T3, T4: These categories represent progressively larger tumor sizes or greater degrees of invasion into nearby tissues.

N: Regional Lymph Nodes
The N category describes the involvement of regional lymph nodes near the primary tumor. Lymph nodes are small, bean-shaped structures that act as filters for lymph fluid, and they are a common site for cancer to spread. The N category uses increasing numbers (e.g., N0, N1, N2, N3) to indicate the extent of lymph node involvement.

N0: No regional lymph node involvement.
N1, N2, N3: These categories represent increasing degrees of regional lymph node involvement, indicating the number and size of affected lymph nodes.

M: Distant Metastasis

The M category indicates whether the cancer has spread to distant organs or tissues beyond the primary tumor site and regional lymph nodes. Metastasis is a critical factor in determining the stage of cancer and the prognosis for the patient.

M0: No distant metastasis.
M1: Distant metastasis is present.

Staging Groups:

The combination of T, N, and M categories results in a stage grouping that classifies the cancer into a specific stage. The stages are typically expressed as stage 0 (in situ) to stage IV (advanced or metastatic). The stage of cancer provides crucial information about its extent, prognosis, and appropriate treatment options.

Importance of TNM Staging:

The TNM staging system is essential for several reasons:

Treatment Planning: The TNM stage helps guide treatment decisions by providing information about the cancer's extent and the appropriate therapies for each stage.

Prognosis Prediction: Staging provides valuable prognostic information, allowing healthcare professionals to estimate a patient's likely outcome and survival rate.

Clinical Trials: TNM staging facilitates the inclusion of patients in appropriate clinical trials, helping researchers study new treatments and therapies for specific stages of cancer.

Communication and Research: The
TNM system allows for standardized
communication among healthcare
providers, ensuring consistency in
describing cancer stages for accurate
comparison and analysis in research
studies.

Overall, the TNM staging system is a
fundamental tool in cancer management,
providing crucial information to guide
treatment decisions and predict patient
outcomes. It is an indispensable
component of cancer care, aiding in
improving patient care and advancing
cancer research.

Histological Grading

Histological grading is a system used to evaluate the microscopic appearance of cancer cells and tissues under a microscope. It is an essential component of cancer diagnosis and staging, providing valuable information about the tumor's characteristics, aggressiveness, and potential for growth and spread. Histological grading is commonly used for solid tumors and helps guide treatment decisions and predict patient outcomes. In this chapter, we will explore the significance of histological grading and its application in cancer diagnosis and treatment.

Purpose of Histological Grading:
The primary purpose of histological grading is to assess the differentiation of cancer cells, which refers to how closely the cancer cells resemble normal cells of the tissue from which the tumor originates. Well-differentiated tumors closely resemble normal cells and tend to grow

more slowly and be less aggressive. In contrast, poorly differentiated tumors show significant abnormalities in cell structure and function and tend to grow more rapidly and be more aggressive.

Grading Scales:
Histological grading is typically performed using one of several established grading scales, the most common of which is the Gleason grading system for prostate cancer and the Nottingham grading system for breast cancer. The grading system may use numbers or descriptive terms to classify tumors into different grades.

For example, the Gleason grading system for prostate cancer uses numbers from 1 to 5 to represent different levels of tumor differentiation, with lower numbers indicating well-differentiated tumors and higher numbers indicating poorly differentiated or undifferentiated tumors. The final Gleason score is the sum of the two most prevalent grades observed in the tumor sample.

Grading Criteria:
The criteria for histological grading vary depending on the type of cancer being evaluated. Pathologists assess several cellular features to determine the tumor grade, including:

Nuclear features: The size, shape, and appearance of the cell nuclei are evaluated. Irregularly shaped and enlarged nuclei are associated with poorly differentiated tumors.

Cell arrangement: The way tumor cells are arranged and organized is considered. Well-differentiated tumors may retain some normal tissue patterns, while poorly differentiated tumors often lack any recognizable tissue structure.

Mitotic activity: The number of actively dividing cells (mitotic figures) is counted. Higher mitotic activity is generally associated with more aggressive tumors.

Clinical Significance:
Histological grading has several clinical implications:

Prognosis Prediction: Tumor grade provides valuable information about the tumor's behavior and likely outcomes. Higher-grade tumors are generally associated with a worse prognosis and a higher risk of recurrence and metastasis.

Treatment Decisions: Histological grading helps guide treatment decisions. Higher-grade tumors may require more aggressive treatment strategies, such as surgery, chemotherapy, or radiation therapy.

Research and Clinical Trials:
Histological grading facilitates the inclusion of patients in appropriate clinical trials and helps researchers study the effectiveness of different treatments for specific tumor grades.

Histological grading is a critical tool in cancer diagnosis and treatment planning. It provides valuable information about the tumor's differentiation and aggressiveness, helping to predict patient outcomes and guide treatment decisions. By understanding the histological grade of a tumor, healthcare professionals can provide more personalized and effective care for cancer patients.

Importance of Staging in Treatment Planning

The staging of cancer is a crucial step in the diagnostic process that involves determining the extent and spread of the disease within the body. Staging provides vital information about the size of the primary tumor, its involvement in nearby tissues and lymph nodes, and the presence or absence of distant metastasis. The information obtained through staging plays a pivotal role in treatment planning and management decisions for cancer patients. In this chapter, we will explore the significance of cancer staging in treatment planning.

Tailoring Treatment Approach: Staging helps oncologists tailor the treatment approach to each individual patient. Different stages of cancer may require distinct treatment strategies to achieve the best possible outcomes. For instance:

Early-Stage Cancer (Stage 0 to I): In the early stages, the tumor is localized and has not spread to distant sites. In many cases, surgical removal of the tumor is the primary treatment. Radiation therapy or targeted therapies may also be considered based on the tumor's characteristics.

Locally Advanced Cancer (Stage II to III): In these stages, the tumor has grown larger and may involve nearby tissues or lymph nodes. Treatment often involves a combination of surgery, radiation therapy, and chemotherapy to target both the primary tumor and any potential remaining cancer cells in the nearby area.

Advanced or Metastatic Cancer (Stage IV): At this stage, the cancer has spread to distant organs or tissues. Treatment aims to manage symptoms, slow the progression of the disease, and improve the patient's quality of life. Systemic therapies such as chemotherapy, immunotherapy, and targeted therapies are commonly used.

Predicting Prognosis:
Staging is a strong predictor of a patient's prognosis or likely outcome. Early-stage cancers are generally associated with a more favorable prognosis, as they have a higher likelihood of being curable with treatment. On the other hand, advanced-stage cancers may have a poorer prognosis due to their increased complexity and spread. Prognosis information guides patient counseling, helps manage expectations, and allows patients to make informed decisions about their treatment options and goals of care.

Guiding Clinical Trials:
Cancer staging also plays a critical role in identifying eligible patients for clinical trials. Clinical trials are research studies that investigate new treatments, therapies, or combinations of treatments. Different clinical trials may be designed to test interventions for specific stages of cancer. Accurate staging helps identify patients who may be suitable candidates for particular clinical trials, providing them

with access to potentially innovative therapies and contributing to the advancement of cancer research.

Monitoring Treatment Response: Staging is not a one-time event but an ongoing process. As patients undergo treatment, their cancer's response to therapy is monitored. Imaging studies and other diagnostic tests are used to reassess the tumor's size and extent, which may lead to changes in the stage. Monitoring treatment response helps healthcare providers modify treatment plans as needed, ensuring that patients receive the most effective and appropriate care throughout their cancer journey.

Cancer staging is an essential component of treatment planning. It guides the selection of appropriate therapies, predicts prognosis, identifies patients for clinical trials, and facilitates ongoing monitoring of treatment response. Accurate staging provides a comprehensive picture of the disease, empowering healthcare teams and

patients to make informed decisions and
optimize cancer care.

81

Surgery: Resection and Debulking

Surgery is one of the primary treatment modalities for cancer and involves the removal of the tumor or affected tissue from the body. Depending on the cancer type, location, stage, and the patient's overall health, surgery may be performed with curative intent to completely remove the cancer or with palliative intent to alleviate symptoms and improve quality of life. Two common surgical approaches used in cancer treatment are resection and debulking.

Resection:
Resection, also known as excision or surgical resection, is a surgical procedure in which the entire tumor or affected tissue is removed from the body, along with a surrounding margin of healthy tissue to ensure complete removal.

The goal of resection is curative, aiming to eliminate all visible cancer cells and prevent local recurrence. Resection is often used in the treatment of solid tumors, such as breast cancer, colorectal cancer, lung cancer, and many others.

There are different types of resection procedures, including:

Lumpectomy: A type of breast-conserving surgery where only the tumor and a small margin of normal breast tissue are removed. Lumpectomy is commonly performed for early-stage breast cancer.

Hemihepatectomy: Surgical removal of one-half of the liver. It may be performed for certain cases of liver cancer or liver metastases.

Segmental or Wedge Resection: Removal of a segment or wedge-shaped portion of an organ, such as the lung or kidney, containing the tumor.

Total or Radical Resection: Removal of the entire organ affected by cancer, such as the removal of the entire breast in a mastectomy or the entire prostate in a radical prostatectomy.

Debulking:
Debulking surgery, also known as cytoreduction, is a surgical procedure in which a portion of a large tumor is removed, but complete resection is not possible due to the tumor's size, location, or spread to surrounding tissues or organs. The primary goal of debulking is palliative, aiming to reduce tumor size and alleviate symptoms such as pain, obstruction, or bleeding. Debulking is commonly used in advanced-stage cancers, where the tumor burden is significant and complete removal is not feasible.

Debulking surgery is often combined with other treatment modalities, such as chemotherapy or radiation therapy, to further control tumor growth and improve the patient's quality of life.

It is important to note that not all cancers are amenable to surgery, and the decision to perform surgery depends on various factors, including the cancer type, stage, location, and the patient's overall health and preferences. In some cases, surgery may be used in combination with other treatments, such as chemotherapy, radiation therapy, immunotherapy, or targeted therapies, to achieve the best possible outcome for the patient.

Overall, surgery plays a critical role in the management of cancer. Resection aims for curative intent by removing the entire tumor, while debulking surgery focuses on palliative care by reducing tumor burden and improving symptoms. Surgical approaches are often part of a comprehensive treatment plan, tailored to each patient's specific cancer type and stage, and may be used in combination with other therapies to optimize cancer care and improve patient outcomes.

Chemotherapy is a systemic cancer treatment that uses drugs to kill or inhibit the growth of rapidly dividing cancer cells throughout the body. It is an essential component of cancer therapy and can be used as a primary treatment, adjuvant therapy (given after primary treatment to reduce the risk of recurrence), neoadjuvant therapy (given before primary treatment to shrink the tumor), or palliative care (to relieve symptoms and improve quality of life). In this chapter, we will explore the principles of chemotherapy and common agents used in cancer treatment.

Principles of Chemotherapy:

Systemic Treatment: Chemotherapy is administered in a way that allows it to enter the bloodstream and circulate throughout the body. This systemic approach is effective in targeting cancer cells that may have spread to other parts of the body, making it suitable for treating metastatic cancer.

Cell Cycle Specificity: Chemotherapy drugs can be categorized as cell cycle-specific or cell cycle-nonspecific. Cell cycle-specific drugs target specific phases of the cell cycle when cancer cells are actively dividing. Cell cycle-nonspecific drugs work throughout the cell cycle and can target both dividing and non-dividing cancer cells.

Combination Therapy: In many cases, chemotherapy is administered as a combination of drugs. Using multiple drugs with different mechanisms of action helps improve treatment effectiveness and reduces the risk of developing drug resistance.

Dosing and Treatment Schedule: Chemotherapy drugs are often given in cycles to allow the body time to recover between treatments. The treatment schedule and dosing may vary depending on the cancer type, stage, and individual patient factors.

Common Chemotherapy Agents:

There are numerous chemotherapy agents used in cancer treatment. Some of the most common types include:

Alkylating Agents: Alkylating agents work by attaching an alkyl group to DNA molecules, disrupting the DNA structure and preventing cancer cells from dividing. Examples include cyclophosphamide, cisplatin, and carboplatin.

Antimetabolites: Antimetabolites interfere with DNA and RNA synthesis by mimicking essential cellular components. They disrupt cancer cell growth and division. Common antimetabolites include methotrexate, 5-fluorouracil (5-FU), and capecitabine.

Anthracyclines: Anthracyclines inhibit DNA and RNA synthesis by intercalating into the DNA strands, causing breaks in the DNA. Doxorubicin and epirubicin are examples of anthracycline drugs.

Taxanes: Taxanes interfere with microtubules, which are essential for cell division. These drugs prevent cancer cells from separating their chromosomes during cell division. Paclitaxel and docetaxel are common taxanes.

Platinum-based Drugs: Platinum-based drugs, such as cisplatin and carboplatin, form crosslinks with DNA, preventing the cancer cells from replicating and dividing.

Vinca Alkaloids: Vinca alkaloids block microtubule formation, hindering cell division. Common vinca alkaloids include vincristine and vinblastine.

Topoisomerase Inhibitors: Topoisomerase inhibitors interfere with the enzymes that control DNA structure during replication. Etoposide and irinotecan are examples of topoisomerase inhibitors.

Targeted Therapies: While not traditional chemotherapy, targeted therapies are a type of systemic treatment that specifically targets cancer cells based on their molecular characteristics. Examples include trastuzumab for HER2-positive breast cancer and imatinib for certain types of leukemia and gastrointestinal stromal tumors (GISTs).

Chemotherapy is a potent treatment that can cause side effects due to its impact on both cancer cells and normal healthy cells. Common side effects include hair loss, nausea, fatigue, and decreased blood cell counts. However, advances in supportive care have improved the management of side effects, making chemotherapy more tolerable for many patients.

The choice of chemotherapy agents and treatment approach is individualized for each patient based on factors such as cancer type, stage, overall health, and treatment goals. Chemotherapy is often used in combination with other treatment modalities, such as surgery, radiation therapy, immunotherapy, or targeted therapies, to achieve the best possible outcomes for cancer patients.

Radiation therapy, also known as radiotherapy, is a localized cancer treatment that uses high-energy beams of radiation to destroy or damage cancer cells. It is a key component of cancer treatment and can be used to shrink tumors, eliminate cancer cells, or alleviate symptoms in both early-stage and advanced cancers. Radiation therapy may be used alone or in combination with other treatment modalities, such as surgery, chemotherapy, or immunotherapy. In this chapter, we will explore the techniques and applications of radiation therapy in cancer treatment.

Techniques of Radiation Therapy:

External Beam Radiation Therapy (EBRT): EBRT is the most common type of radiation therapy. It involves delivering radiation to the tumor from outside the body using a machine called a linear accelerator. The patient typically lies on a treatment table, and the radiation is precisely targeted at the tumor to spare surrounding healthy tissues. EBRT is usually administered daily over several weeks, with each session lasting a few minutes.

Intensity-Modulated Radiation Therapy (IMRT): IMRT is an advanced form of external beam radiation that uses computer-controlled beams to deliver varying intensities of radiation to different parts of the tumor. This technique allows for more precise targeting of the tumor, reducing radiation exposure to nearby healthy tissues and potentially minimizing side effects.

Stereotactic Body Radiation Therapy (SBRT): SBRT delivers highly focused and high-dose radiation to the tumor in a few treatment sessions. It is commonly used for small, well-defined tumors in areas where precision is critical, such as the lung, liver, and spine.

Brachytherapy: Brachytherapy, also known as internal radiation therapy, involves placing a radioactive source directly inside or very close to the tumor. This allows for a higher dose of radiation to be delivered to the tumor while minimizing exposure to surrounding healthy tissues. Brachytherapy is commonly used in gynecological cancers, prostate cancer, and some head and neck cancers.

Applications of Radiation Therapy:

Curative Intent: Radiation therapy can be used with curative intent to treat localized tumors or early-stage cancers. It aims to eradicate the cancer cells completely and achieve long-term remission.

Adjuvant Therapy: In cases where cancer has been surgically removed, adjuvant radiation therapy may be given to eliminate any remaining cancer cells and reduce the risk of local recurrence.

Neoadjuvant Therapy: Neoadjuvant radiation therapy is administered before surgery to shrink the tumor and make it more manageable for surgical removal.

Palliative Care: For advanced-stage cancers or metastatic disease, radiation therapy can be used palliatively to relieve symptoms such as pain, bleeding, or obstruction, and improve the patient's quality of life.

Combined Modality Treatment: Radiation therapy is often used in combination with other treatment modalities, such as chemotherapy or targeted therapies, to enhance treatment effectiveness and improve outcomes.

Benefits and Side Effects:
Radiation therapy offers several benefits, including precise tumor targeting, non-invasiveness, and the ability to preserve organ function. The treatment is generally well-tolerated, and side effects are often limited to the treated area. Common side effects may include fatigue, skin irritation, and changes in the treated area.

However, radiation therapy can also cause long-term side effects, depending on the location and dose of radiation delivered. Healthcare providers carefully consider the risks and benefits of radiation therapy for each individual patient and develop personalized treatment plans to optimize outcomes and minimize side effects.

Radiation therapy is a valuable and versatile treatment option in the fight against cancer. With different techniques and applications, radiation therapy is used for curative purposes, adjuvant or neoadjuvant treatments, palliative care, and in combination with other therapies.

By harnessing the power of radiation to target and destroy cancer cells, radiation therapy plays a critical role in improving the quality of life and prognosis for many cancer patients.

Chapter 7: Targeted Therapies

Immunotherapy: Harnessing the Immune System against Cancer

Immunotherapy is a revolutionary approach to cancer treatment that harnesses the body's own immune system to recognize and attack cancer cells. Unlike traditional treatments like surgery, chemotherapy, and radiation therapy, which directly target cancer cells, immunotherapy works by stimulating the immune system to recognize cancer cells as foreign invaders and mount an immune response against them. This innovative form of cancer therapy has shown remarkable success in treating various types of cancer and has transformed the landscape of cancer treatment. In this chapter, we will explore the principles of immunotherapy and its applications in cancer treatment.

Principles of Immunotherapy:

Immune Recognition: Cancer cells can often evade detection by the immune system because they arise from the body's own cells and display certain molecules that prevent immune cells from recognizing them as foreign. Immunotherapy uses various strategies to help immune cells recognize cancer cells as abnormal and target them for destruction.

Immune Activation: Immunotherapy aims to activate and boost the activity of specific immune cells, such as T cells and natural killer (NK) cells, which are responsible for recognizing and destroying cancer cells. This can be achieved through the administration of immune-stimulating substances, such as cytokines or immune checkpoint inhibitors.

Immune Checkpoint Blockade: Cancer cells can exploit certain "checkpoint" molecules on immune cells to evade attack.

Immunotherapy can block these checkpoints, such as programmed cell death protein 1 (PD-1) and cytotoxic T-lymphocyte-associated protein 4 (CTLA-4), to unleash the immune system's ability to target cancer cells more effectively.

Applications of Immunotherapy:

Checkpoint Inhibitors: Checkpoint inhibitors are a common form of immunotherapy that has shown significant success in various cancer types. Drugs like pembrolizumab, nivolumab, and ipilimumab target the PD-1 and CTLA-4 checkpoints, helping T cells recognize and attack cancer cells. Checkpoint inhibitors have been particularly effective in treating melanoma, lung cancer, kidney cancer, bladder cancer, and certain types of lymphoma and head and neck cancers.

CAR T-cell Therapy: Chimeric antigen receptor (CAR) T-cell therapy is a personalized form of immunotherapy that involves modifying a patient's own T cells to express a specific receptor (CAR) that targets cancer cells. The modified CAR T cells are then infused back into the patient's bloodstream to seek out and destroy cancer cells. CAR T-cell therapy has shown remarkable success in treating certain types of blood cancers, such as acute lymphoblastic leukemia (ALL) and certain types of non-Hodgkin lymphoma.

Cancer Vaccines: Cancer vaccines are designed to stimulate the immune system to recognize and attack cancer cells. They can be made from cancer cells, proteins, or genetic material. Cancer vaccines are being developed for various cancer types, including prostate cancer, melanoma, and certain types of brain cancer.

Adoptive T-cell Therapy: Adoptive T-cell therapy involves extracting T cells from a patient, engineering them to recognize cancer cells, and then expanding their numbers in the laboratory. These engineered T cells are then infused back into the patient to target and destroy cancer cells.

Benefits and Side Effects:

Immunotherapy has shown remarkable benefits in certain cancer patients, leading to prolonged remissions and even cures in some cases. Unlike traditional treatments, immunotherapy offers the potential for long-lasting responses and can be effective in cancers that have become resistant to other therapies. Additionally, immunotherapy tends to have fewer side effects than chemotherapy and radiation therapy, as it specifically targets cancer cells without damaging normal cells.

However, not all patients respond equally to immunotherapy, and the success of treatment depends on factors such as the type of cancer, the stage of the disease, and the individual's overall health. Immunotherapy can cause immune-related side effects, which occur when the immune system attacks normal tissues in addition to cancer cells. These side effects can affect various organs and may include skin rash, diarrhea, inflammation of the lungs (pneumonitis), and others. Prompt recognition and management of these side effects are crucial for ensuring the safety and efficacy of immunotherapy.

Immunotherapy represents a groundbreaking advancement in cancer treatment by empowering the body's immune system to fight cancer. It has demonstrated remarkable success in various cancer types and offers new hope for patients with advanced or previously treatment-resistant cancers. As research continues to advance, immunotherapy is likely to play an increasingly prominent role in cancer care, offering more personalized and effective treatment options for patients in the future.

Monoclonal Antibodies and Immune Checkpoint Inhibitors

Monoclonal antibodies and immune checkpoint inhibitors are two important classes of immunotherapy that have revolutionized cancer treatment. Both approaches harness the power of the immune system to target and destroy cancer cells, but they work through different mechanisms. In this chapter, we will explore the principles of monoclonal antibodies and immune checkpoint inhibitors and their applications in cancer therapy.

Monoclonal Antibodies (mAbs): Monoclonal antibodies are lab-created antibodies designed to target specific proteins on the surface of cancer cells. These antibodies are engineered to recognize and bind to these target proteins, leading to a series of immune responses that can directly or indirectly kill cancer cells.

There are different types of monoclonal antibodies used in cancer treatment, each with distinct mechanisms of action:

Antibodies that directly target cancer cells: Some monoclonal antibodies carry a toxic payload or a radioactive substance that is released upon binding to the cancer cell. This effectively delivers a cytotoxic agent directly to the tumor cells.

Antibodies that block cell signaling: Certain monoclonal antibodies interfere with the signaling pathways that promote cancer cell growth and survival. By blocking these pathways, they inhibit cancer cell proliferation and induce cell death.

Antibodies that trigger immune response: Some monoclonal antibodies bind to cancer cells and recruit immune cells to attack and destroy the cancer cells. These immune cells can include T cells, natural killer (NK) cells, and macrophages.

Examples of monoclonal antibodies used in cancer treatment include:

Trastuzumab (Herceptin): Used for HER2-positive breast cancer and gastric cancer.

Rituximab (Rituxan): Used for certain types of non-Hodgkin lymphoma and chronic lymphocytic leukemia (CLL).

Bevacizumab (Avastin): Used for various cancers to inhibit the growth of blood vessels that supply tumors.

Cetuximab (Erbitux) and panitumumab (Vectibix): Used for colorectal cancer and certain head and neck cancers.

Immune Checkpoint Inhibitors:45680 Immune checkpoint inhibitors are a class of immunotherapy drugs that target specific molecules on immune cells, called checkpoints, to enhance the immune system's ability to recognize and attack cancer cells. These checkpoints normally serve as "brakes" on the immune response to prevent excessive immune reactions and maintain immune system balance. Cancer cells often exploit these checkpoints to evade immune detection. Immune checkpoint inhibitors block these checkpoints, releasing the "brakes" and allowing the immune system to mount a more potent anti-cancer response.

The two most commonly targeted immune checkpoints are programmed cell death protein 1 (PD-1) and cytotoxic T-lymphocyte-associated protein 4 (CTLA-4). PD-1 inhibitors, such as pembrolizumab (Keytruda) and nivolumab (Opdivo), are used in various cancers, including melanoma, lung cancer, kidney cancer, bladder cancer, and others. CTLA-4 inhibitors, such as ipilimumab (Yervoy), are mainly used for advanced melanoma.

Applications and Combination Therapy: Monoclonal antibodies and immune checkpoint inhibitors have shown significant success in the treatment of various cancers, both as standalone treatments and in combination with other therapies. They have been effective in achieving long-lasting responses and even cures in some cases, particularly in cancers that were previously considered difficult to treat.

Combination therapy with these immunotherapies and other treatment modalities, such as chemotherapy and targeted therapies, is becoming increasingly common. This approach aims to enhance treatment effectiveness by targeting cancer cells through multiple mechanisms, overcoming potential resistance, and improving overall patient outcomes.

Benefits and Side Effects:
Monoclonal antibodies and immune checkpoint inhibitors have several benefits, including targeted action against cancer cells, potential for durable responses, and lower toxicity compared to traditional treatments like chemotherapy. However, they can also cause immune-related side effects, which occur when the immune system attacks normal tissues in addition to cancer cells.

These side effects can affect various organs and may include skin rash, diarrhea, inflammation of the lungs (pneumonitis), and others. Early recognition and management of these side effects are crucial to ensuring the safety and efficacy of immunotherapy.

Monoclonal antibodies and immune checkpoint inhibitors are groundbreaking therapies that have transformed cancer treatment by harnessing the body's immune system to fight cancer. Their success in various cancers highlights the potential for immunotherapy to revolutionize cancer care and provide new hope for patients with advanced or previously treatment-resistant cancers. As research in immunotherapy continues, these treatments are likely to play an increasingly prominent role in cancer therapy and lead to further advancements in personalized and targeted cancer treatment.

Personalized medicine and precision oncology are cutting-edge approaches to cancer treatment that aim to tailor medical decisions and therapies to individual patients based on their unique characteristics, genetic makeup, and molecular profile. These approaches recognize that each person's cancer is distinct and that the most effective treatment may vary from patient to patient. Personalized medicine and precision oncology have revolutionized cancer care by improving treatment outcomes, reducing side effects, and optimizing the overall management of the disease.

Principles of Personalized Medicine and Precision Oncology:

Molecular Profiling: Personalized medicine and precision oncology rely on advanced technologies that allow comprehensive molecular profiling of a patient's tumor. These profiles identify specific genetic mutations, alterations, or biomarkers that drive the growth and spread of the cancer.

Targeted Therapies: With the knowledge gained from molecular profiling, targeted therapies can be selected. Targeted therapies are drugs designed to specifically target the molecular alterations present in the cancer cells, while sparing healthy cells. This approach increases treatment effectiveness and reduces the risk of side effects compared to traditional therapies.

Biomarker-Driven Treatment: Biomarkers, which can be genetic, molecular, or cellular, provide crucial information about a patient's response to treatment and prognosis. Personalized medicine uses these biomarkers to guide treatment decisions, predict treatment outcomes, and monitor treatment response over time.

Individualized Treatment Plans:
Personalized medicine aims to create individualized treatment plans based on the specific characteristics of a patient's cancer. Treatment options may include a combination of surgery, radiation therapy, chemotherapy, immunotherapy, and targeted therapies, customized to achieve the best possible outcome for that patient.

Applications of Personalized Medicine and Precision Oncology:

Targeted Therapies: Precision oncology has led to the development of numerous targeted therapies that are designed to inhibit specific molecules or pathways that drive cancer growth. These therapies have shown significant success in various cancer types, such as HER2-targeted therapies in breast cancer and EGFR inhibitors in lung cancer.

Genomic Profiling: Advances in genomic profiling techniques have enabled the identification of specific genetic mutations and alterations associated with different cancers. This information guides treatment decisions and can help match patients with clinical trials investigating new targeted therapies.

Liquid Biopsies: Liquid biopsies are a non-invasive method of obtaining genetic information about a tumor through a blood sample. This approach allows for real-time monitoring of treatment response and the detection of potential resistance mechanisms.

Companion Diagnostics: Companion diagnostics are tests that identify biomarkers that predict whether a patient is likely to respond to a specific treatment. They are crucial in guiding the use of targeted therapies to patients who are most likely to benefit from them.

Benefits and Future Perspectives:

The benefits of personalized medicine and precision oncology are significant and multifaceted:

Improved Treatment Outcomes: By targeting the specific genetic and molecular alterations driving a patient's cancer, targeted therapies have shown remarkable efficacy and improved treatment outcomes.

Reduced Side Effects: Precision oncology minimizes damage to healthy cells, leading to reduced side effects compared to traditional treatments.

Enhanced Clinical Trial Design: Molecular profiling and biomarker-driven approaches allow for more effective and efficient clinical trial designs, leading to faster drug development and approval processes.

Evolution of Treatment: Personalized medicine is continually evolving as new genetic and molecular insights are discovered. This dynamic field holds the promise of continuously improving cancer care with more effective and less toxic treatments.

Despite its success, challenges remain in implementing personalized medicine and precision oncology on a broader scale. These challenges include access to advanced technologies, the need for collaboration between various stakeholders, and the integration of large-scale genomic data into clinical practice.

Personalized medicine and precision oncology represent a paradigm shift in cancer treatment, moving away from a one-size-fits-all approach to an individualized and targeted strategy. By utilizing molecular profiling, targeted therapies, and biomarker-driven treatment decisions, personalized medicine has transformed cancer care, offering patients more effective treatments and better quality of life. As research and technology continue to advance, the future of personalized medicine holds great promise in further improving cancer outcomes and revolutionizing cancer care on a global scale.

Chapter 8: Emerging and Experimental Cancer Therapies

Gene Therapy: Engineering Cells to Fight Cancer

Gene therapy is an innovative and promising approach to cancer treatment that involves the modification of a patient's own cells to enhance their ability to recognize and fight cancer. This cutting-edge therapy aims to correct genetic defects, boost the immune system, or directly target cancer cells, offering a personalized and targeted treatment approach. Gene therapy has the potential to revolutionize cancer treatment by providing more effective and long-lasting responses, with fewer side effects compared to traditional treatments. In this chapter, we will explore the principles of gene therapy and its applications in fighting cancer.

Principles of Gene Therapy:

Genetic Modification: Gene therapy involves the transfer of genetic material into a patient's cells to correct or alter their genetic makeup. This can be achieved using various delivery systems, such as viral vectors or non-viral methods, to introduce therapeutic genes into the cells.

Targeting Cancer Cells: Gene therapy can be designed to directly target cancer cells by introducing genes that induce cell death, inhibit cancer growth, or sensitize cancer cells to other treatments.

Enhancing the Immune Response: Gene therapy can also be used to enhance the patient's immune response against cancer cells. For example, chimeric antigen receptor (CAR) T-cell therapy is a form of gene therapy that involves modifying the patient's T cells to express a receptor that targets cancer cells.

Applications of Gene Therapy in Cancer Treatment:

CAR T-Cell Therapy: CAR T-cell therapy is a groundbreaking form of gene therapy that involves extracting a patient's T cells, genetically engineering them to express a specific receptor that targets cancer cells, and then infusing these modified CAR T cells back into the patient's bloodstream. Once inside the body, the CAR T cells seek out and destroy cancer cells that express the targeted antigen. CAR T-cell therapy has shown remarkable success in treating certain types of blood cancers, such as acute lymphoblastic leukemia (ALL) and certain types of non-Hodgkin lymphoma.

Tumor Suppressor Gene Therapy: Tumor suppressor genes are genes that normally help regulate cell growth and prevent cancer formation. In gene therapy, the missing or defective tumor suppressor gene can be replaced or restored in cancer cells to inhibit their growth and promote cell death.

Oncolytic Viruses: Oncolytic viruses are genetically engineered viruses that selectively infect and replicate within cancer cells, causing their destruction. These viruses can also stimulate the immune system to recognize and attack cancer cells more effectively.

Immune Modulation: Gene therapy can be used to modify immune cells to enhance their activity against cancer cells. For example, genes that enhance the activity of natural killer (NK) cells or other immune cells can be introduced to improve their cancer-killing capabilities.

Benefits and Challenges:
Gene therapy offers several potential benefits for cancer treatment:

Precise Targeting: Gene therapy can specifically target cancer cells while sparing healthy cells, reducing the risk of side effects associated with traditional treatments.

Long-Lasting Response: Gene therapy has the potential to provide long-lasting responses and even cures, especially in patients with limited treatment options.

Personalized Treatment: Gene therapy can be tailored to each patient's specific cancer type and genetic makeup, offering personalized and targeted treatment strategies.

However, gene therapy also faces some challenges, including:

Safety Concerns: The use of viral vectors and genetic modification carries safety risks, including the potential for unintended side effects or immune responses.

High Cost: Gene therapy is currently a complex and expensive treatment, limiting its accessibility to many patients.

Research and Development: Continued research and development are needed to optimize gene therapy approaches, improve safety, and expand its applications to various cancer types.

Gene therapy is an exciting frontier in cancer treatment that holds great promise in improving patient outcomes and transforming cancer care. By engineering cells to target and fight cancer, gene therapy offers a personalized and precise approach to cancer treatment. As research and technology continue to advance, gene therapy is expected to play an increasingly significant role in the future of cancer therapy, providing new hope for patients with challenging and previously untreatable cancers.

Nanotechnology in Cancer Treatment

Nanotechnology in cancer treatment is an emerging field that utilizes tiny particles, known as nanoparticles, to target and deliver therapeutic agents specifically to cancer cells. These nanoparticles are engineered to have unique properties that allow them to circulate in the bloodstream, evade the immune system, and selectively accumulate in tumor tissues. Nanotechnology has the potential to revolutionize cancer treatment by improving the effectiveness of therapies, reducing side effects, and enabling more precise and personalized treatment strategies.

Principles of Nanotechnology in Cancer Treatment:

Targeted Drug Delivery: Nanoparticles can be loaded with chemotherapy drugs, immunotherapies, or other therapeutic agents.

Due to their small size and surface modifications, these nanoparticles can selectively accumulate in tumor tissues, delivering the therapeutic payload directly to cancer cells while sparing healthy cells.

Enhanced Permeability and Retention Effect (EPR): Tumor tissues often have leaky blood vessels, allowing nanoparticles to passively accumulate in the tumor through the EPR effect. This phenomenon allows nanoparticles to accumulate preferentially in tumor tissues and remain there for an extended period, enhancing drug delivery and efficacy.

Multifunctional Nanoparticles: Nanoparticles can be designed to have multiple functions, such as combining diagnostic imaging and therapy in a single agent. These multifunctional nanoparticles can help with early cancer detection, treatment planning, and monitoring treatment response.

Overcoming Drug Resistance:
Nanotechnology can help overcome drug
resistance by delivering combination
therapies or targeting specific drug-
resistant pathways in cancer cells.

**Applications of Nanotechnology in
Cancer Treatment**:

Targeted Drug Delivery: Nanoparticles
can deliver chemotherapy drugs directly to
the tumor site, reducing off-target effects
and improving the therapeutic index of
these drugs.

Photodynamic Therapy (PDT): In PDT,
nanoparticles are used to deliver
photosensitizing agents to cancer cells.
When exposed to light of a specific
wavelength, the photosensitizing agents
generate reactive oxygen species, causing
localized damage and cell death in the
tumor.

Hyperthermia: Nanoparticles can also be used to induce localized hyperthermia (elevated temperature) in tumor tissues. This heat-based treatment can help destroy cancer cells while sparing surrounding healthy tissues.

Imaging: Nanoparticles can be labeled with contrast agents, enabling their use in various imaging techniques, such as magnetic resonance imaging (MRI), computed tomography (CT), and positron emission tomography (PET). This allows for non-invasive tumor visualization and improved cancer diagnosis and staging.

Benefits and Challenges:
Nanotechnology offers several benefits in cancer treatment:

Enhanced Drug Delivery: Nanoparticles improve drug delivery to tumor tissues, increasing treatment effectiveness and reducing side effects on healthy tissues.

Precision and Personalization:
Nanotechnology enables more precise and
personalized treatment approaches,
tailoring therapies to individual patients
based on their specific cancer type and
molecular profile.

Combination Therapies: Nanoparticles
can deliver multiple therapeutic agents
simultaneously, allowing for combination
therapies and overcoming drug resistance.

*However, challenges remain in the
clinical translation and widespread
adoption of nanotechnology in cancer
treatment*:
Safety Concerns: The long-term safety of
nanoparticles in humans is still under
investigation, and potential toxicities and
side effects need to be thoroughly assessed.

Manufacturing Complexity: The
production of nanoparticles with precise
characteristics and reproducibility can be
challenging and may impact their
scalability and cost.

Regulatory Approval: Regulatory approval processes for nanotechnology-based therapies require rigorous evaluation to ensure their safety and efficacy.

Nanotechnology is a promising and rapidly evolving field in cancer treatment. By enabling targeted drug delivery, enhancing imaging capabilities, and offering multifunctional therapeutic options, nanotechnology has the potential to revolutionize cancer care and improve patient outcomes. Continued research, technological advancements, and collaborations between academia, industry, and regulatory agencies are essential to realizing the full potential of nanotechnology in the fight against cancer. As this field progresses, nanotechnology is expected to play an increasingly significant role in the future of cancer treatment and contribute to more effective and personalized therapies for cancer patients.

Hyperthermia and photodynamic therapy (PDT) are two distinct therapeutic approaches used in cancer treatment, both of which aim to selectively target and destroy cancer cells while minimizing damage to surrounding healthy tissues. These therapies offer promising strategies for enhancing the effectiveness of cancer treatment and have been explored in various cancer types.

Hyperthermia:
Hyperthermia is a treatment that involves raising the temperature of tumor tissues to induce localized heating. This elevated temperature can cause cell death, either directly by damaging cancer cells or indirectly by enhancing the effects of other cancer treatments, such as radiation therapy or chemotherapy.

Principles of Hyperthermia:

Localized Heating: Hyperthermia involves carefully raising the temperature of the tumor region, typically to a range of 41-45 degrees Celsius (105-113 degrees Fahrenheit). This temperature range is chosen because it is cytotoxic to cancer cells while preserving surrounding normal tissues.

Sensitization of Cancer Cells: Hyperthermia can sensitize cancer cells to the effects of radiation or certain chemotherapy drugs, making the tumor more susceptible to these treatments. It disrupts the repair mechanisms of cancer cells, making them more vulnerable to subsequent therapies.

Immune Response: Hyperthermia can also trigger an immune response, stimulating the body's immune system to recognize and attack cancer cells more effectively.

Applications of Hyperthermia:

Combined with Radiation Therapy:
Hyperthermia is often used as an adjunct
to radiation therapy (thermoradiotherapy)
to enhance radiation's effectiveness in
killing cancer cells. Hyperthermia can
increase the sensitivity of cancer cells to
radiation and improve tumor control rates.

Combined with Chemotherapy:
Hyperthermia can be combined with
certain chemotherapy agents to enhance
their effects. By increasing blood flow to
the tumor and disrupting cell repair
mechanisms, hyperthermia can increase
the uptake and efficacy of chemotherapy
drugs.

Localized Hyperthermia: In some cases,
hyperthermia can be delivered locally
through techniques such as radiofrequency
ablation or microwave ablation. These
methods use heat to destroy tumors in
specific locations, such as in liver or lung
cancer.

Photodynamic Therapy (PDT):
PDT is a treatment that uses a combination of light and a photosensitizing agent to selectively destroy cancer cells. The photosensitizing agent is administered to the patient, and when exposed to light of a specific wavelength, it becomes activated and generates reactive oxygen species. These reactive oxygen species cause localized damage to cancer cells, leading to their destruction.

Principles of Photodynamic Therapy:

Selective Activation: The photosensitizing agent is designed to preferentially accumulate in cancer cells. When exposed to light of the appropriate wavelength, the photosensitizer becomes activated and selectively destroys the cancer cells while sparing healthy tissues.

Dual Mechanism: PDT works through both direct cytotoxic effects on cancer cells and indirect effects on the tumor microenvironment, including damage to blood vessels and stimulation of the immune system.

Applications of Photodynamic Therapy:

Localized Treatment: PDT is suitable for treating surface or near-surface tumors, such as skin cancers and certain types of early-stage cancers in the esophagus and lungs.

Palliative Care: PDT can also be used to alleviate symptoms in advanced-stage cancers, such as obstructing tumors in the airways or gastrointestinal tract.

Benefits and Challenges:
Hyperthermia and photodynamic therapy offer several benefits in cancer treatment:

Selective Targeting: Both therapies selectively target and destroy cancer cells, reducing damage to surrounding healthy tissues.

Combined Therapies: Hyperthermia and PDT can be used in combination with other cancer treatments to enhance their efficacy.

Localized Treatment: Both therapies are amenable to localized treatment, allowing for targeted therapy delivery.

Challenges include the need for optimal treatment planning, ensuring appropriate light penetration for PDT, and improving patient selection for hyperthermia treatment.

Hyperthermia and photodynamic therapy are promising and innovative treatment approaches in cancer therapy. By exploiting the selective targeting of cancer cells, these therapies offer the potential to improve treatment outcomes while minimizing side effects. Continued research and clinical trials are needed to further explore and optimize these therapies for different cancer types and in combination with other treatment modalities. As technology and knowledge continue to advance, hyperthermia and PDT are expected to play an increasingly important role in the comprehensive management of cancer.

Chapter 9: Palliative Care and Supportive Intervention

Managing Symptoms and Side Effects

Managing symptoms and side effects is a crucial aspect of cancer care that focuses on providing relief and improving the quality of life for cancer patients. Cancer and its treatments can cause various physical, emotional, and psychological side effects that can be challenging for patients to cope with. An effective symptom management plan involves a multidisciplinary approach, including medical interventions, supportive care, and addressing the emotional and psychological needs of patients and their families.

Common Symptoms and Side Effects:

Pain: Pain is a common symptom experienced by cancer patients, either due to the cancer itself or as a side effect of treatments. Managing pain effectively is essential for improving patients' comfort and well-being.

Fatigue: Cancer-related fatigue is a pervasive and overwhelming tiredness that significantly impacts a patient's ability to function. It can result from the cancer itself, treatments, or other factors related to the disease.

Nausea and Vomiting: Chemotherapy and certain other cancer treatments can cause nausea and vomiting, which can be distressing for patients.

Loss of Appetite and Weight Changes: Cancer and its treatments can lead to a loss of appetite, taste changes, and weight loss, affecting a patient's nutritional status and overall health.

Hair Loss: Some cancer treatments, particularly chemotherapy, can lead to hair loss, which can have emotional and psychological effects on patients.

Cognitive Changes (Chemo Brain): Patients undergoing chemotherapy may experience cognitive changes, such as memory problems and difficulty concentrating, known as chemo brain.

Emotional and Psychological Distress: The cancer journey can evoke a range of emotions, including anxiety, depression, fear, and uncertainty. Emotional and psychological support is essential for patients and their families.

Management Strategies:

Medications: Medications are often prescribed to manage symptoms like pain, nausea, and fatigue. Analgesics, antiemetics, and other supportive medications can significantly improve a patient's comfort.

Palliative Care: Palliative care focuses on providing relief from symptoms and improving the quality of life for patients with serious illnesses, including cancer. Palliative care teams work alongside oncologists to manage symptoms and provide emotional support.

Nutritional Support: Registered dietitians can work with patients to address nutritional needs and manage eating-related challenges during and after cancer treatment.

Physical Activity: Engaging in regular physical activity, as tolerated, can help manage fatigue and improve overall well-being.

Supportive Therapies: Complementary and alternative therapies, such as acupuncture, massage, and relaxation techniques, may help manage symptoms and improve well-being.

Counseling and Support Groups:
Psychosocial support, including
counseling and support groups, can
provide emotional support and help
patients and families cope with the
challenges of cancer.

Survivorship Care: After cancer
treatment, survivors may continue to
experience long-term side effects and
emotional concerns. Survivorship care
plans can help monitor and manage these
issues.

The Role of Communication:
Effective communication between patients,
caregivers, and healthcare providers is
essential for symptom management.
Patients should be encouraged to
communicate openly about their
symptoms and side effects, allowing
healthcare providers to tailor management
strategies accordingly.

Healthcare teams can help set realistic expectations, educate patients about potential side effects, and empower them to actively participate in their care.

Managing symptoms and side effects is an integral part of comprehensive cancer care. A patient-centered approach that addresses physical, emotional, and psychological needs can significantly improve the quality of life for cancer patients. By providing personalized and supportive care, healthcare teams can help patients navigate through their cancer journey with greater comfort, understanding, and resilience.

Psychological and Emotional Support for Patients and Families

Psychological and emotional support for patients and families is a crucial aspect of cancer care that focuses on addressing the emotional and psychological challenges that arise during the cancer journey. A cancer diagnosis can be overwhelming and emotionally distressing, not only for the patient but also for their loved ones. Providing effective support and counseling can help patients and families cope with the psychological impact of cancer, enhance their well-being, and improve their overall quality of life.

Importance of Psychological and Emotional Support:

Coping with Diagnosis and Treatment: A cancer diagnosis can bring about a range of emotions, including fear, anxiety, sadness, and uncertainty. Emotional support helps patients and families navigate these emotions and adjust to the changes brought on by the diagnosis and treatment.

Reducing Stress and Anxiety: Cancer and its treatment can be stressful and anxiety-inducing. Emotional support and counseling can help patients develop coping strategies and relaxation techniques to manage stress and anxiety effectively.

Improving Treatment Adherence: Psychological support can enhance patients' motivation and resilience, leading to improved treatment adherence and better treatment outcomes.

Enhancing Quality of Life: Emotional support can improve the overall quality of life for patients and their families by addressing emotional distress and fostering a sense of hope and well-being.

Psychological and Emotional Support Services:

Oncology Social Workers: Oncology social workers are trained professionals who provide counseling, support, and resources to cancer patients and their families. They can assist with emotional coping, financial concerns, and access to support services.

Psychologists and Psychiatrists: Mental health professionals, such as psychologists and psychiatrists, can provide counseling, psychotherapy, and psychiatric support for patients and families dealing with emotional distress and psychological challenges.

Support Groups: Cancer support groups offer a safe space for patients and families to share their experiences, exchange support, and learn from others facing similar challenges.

Art Therapy and Mindfulness Programs: Creative expression through art therapy and mindfulness programs can help patients manage stress, anxiety, and emotional challenges.

Palliative Care and Hospice Teams: Palliative care and hospice teams provide specialized support for patients with advanced or terminal cancer, focusing on symptom management, emotional support, and end-of-life care.

Online Resources: Online platforms and websites provide information, resources, and forums for patients and families seeking support and connection with others in similar situations.

The Role of Communication and Family Support:
Effective communication between patients, families, and healthcare providers is vital in providing emotional support. Family members play a crucial role in offering emotional support to the patient during

their cancer journey. Their involvement can strengthen the patient's emotional resilience and help them feel cared for and understood.

Family members should be encouraged to express their emotions and concerns openly and seek their own support through counseling or support groups, as caregiving can also be emotionally challenging.

Psychological and emotional support is a fundamental component of comprehensive cancer care. Addressing the emotional well-being of patients and families is essential in helping them navigate the challenges of cancer diagnosis and treatment. By providing counseling, support, and resources, healthcare teams can foster emotional resilience and improve the overall well-being and quality of life for cancer patients and their families.

End-of-Life Care and Hospice

End-of-life care and hospice are specialized forms of care that focus on providing comfort, support, and dignity to patients with advanced, life-limiting illnesses, including cancer, during the last stages of their life. The primary goal of end-of-life care and hospice is to ensure that patients experience the best possible quality of life while managing symptoms and providing emotional and spiritual support for both the patient and their loved ones.

Key Principles of End-of-Life Care and Hospice:

Palliative Approach: End-of-life care and hospice adopt a palliative care approach, which means that the focus is on relieving pain and managing symptoms to provide comfort rather than trying to cure the underlying illness.

Patient-Centered Care: Care is tailored to meet the unique needs and preferences of each patient. The patient's wishes and goals are central to decision-making, ensuring that their preferences for care and treatment are respected.

Multidisciplinary Care: A team of healthcare professionals, including physicians, nurses, social workers, chaplains, and other specialists, work collaboratively to address the physical, emotional, spiritual, and social needs of the patient and their family.

Emotional and Psychological Support: End-of-life care and hospice provide emotional and psychological support to both the patient and their family members, acknowledging the challenges and emotional distress that arise during this time.

Bereavement Support: Hospice programs often provide bereavement support to the family and loved ones after the patient's death, offering counseling and resources to help them cope with their grief.

Services and Support Provided:

Pain and Symptom Management: Controlling pain and managing distressing symptoms are central to end-of-life care. Medications and other interventions are used to alleviate physical discomfort and promote comfort.

Emotional and Spiritual Support: Hospice care addresses the emotional and spiritual needs of the patient and their family members, providing counseling and spiritual guidance as requested.

Assistance with Daily Living Activities: Hospice teams may provide assistance with activities of daily living, such as bathing, dressing, and eating, to support the patient's comfort and well-being.

Respite Care: Hospice programs may offer respite care services, giving family caregivers a temporary break to rest and take care of themselves.

24/7 Availability: Hospice care is available around the clock, ensuring that patients and families have access to support and care whenever needed.

Advanced Care Planning: Hospice teams assist patients in making decisions about their care and treatment preferences, including the use of life-sustaining treatments, based on their values and goals.

Eligibility and Timing:
Eligibility for hospice care typically requires a prognosis of six months or less if the illness follows its expected course. However, hospice care can be provided for longer periods if needed, as long as the patient continues to meet the eligibility criteria.

The decision to enter hospice care is based on the patient's medical condition and their goals and wishes for care. It is essential for patients and families to have open discussions with their healthcare team about end-of-life care options.

End-of-life care and hospice play a critical role in providing compassionate and supportive care to patients with advanced, life-limiting illnesses and their families. By focusing on comfort, symptom management, and emotional support, these specialized forms of care ensure that patients experience dignity and respect during the final stages of life. Hospice care emphasizes the importance of quality of life and allows patients and their families to spend meaningful time together, making the end-of-life journey as comfortable and meaningful as possible.

Chapter 10: Cancer Prevention and Future Outlook

Lifestyle Modifications and Cancer Prevention

Lifestyle modifications play a significant role in cancer prevention, as certain lifestyle factors have been associated with an increased risk of developing various types of cancer. Making healthy lifestyle choices can help reduce the risk of cancer and promote overall well-being. While not all cancers can be prevented, adopting a health-conscious lifestyle can contribute to a lower cancer risk and improve overall health outcomes. Here are some key lifestyle modifications that can help in cancer prevention:

Avoid Tobacco and Limit Alcohol Consumption:
Tobacco use, including smoking and smokeless tobacco, is one of the most

significant risk factors for cancer. Quitting smoking and avoiding tobacco products can significantly lower the risk of developing lung, oral, throat, and other cancers.
Limiting alcohol consumption is also essential, as excessive alcohol intake is linked to an increased risk of certain cancers, including those of the liver, breast, esophagus, and mouth. Reducing alcohol consumption can decrease cancer risk.

Maintain a Healthy Diet:
A balanced diet rich in fruits, vegetables, whole grains, and lean proteins is associated with a lower risk of cancer. These foods are high in vitamins, minerals, antioxidants, and fiber, which have cancer-protective properties.
Limit the consumption of processed and red meats, as high intake has been linked to an increased risk of certain cancers, particularly colorectal cancer.

Achieve and Maintain a Healthy Weight:
Being overweight or obese is a risk factor
for several cancers, including breast, colon,
kidney, and endometrial cancers.
Adopting a healthy eating plan and
engaging in regular physical activity can
help achieve and maintain a healthy
weight.

Engage in Regular Physical Activity:
Regular physical activity is associated
with a reduced risk of several cancers,
including breast, colon, and endometrial
cancers. Aim for at least 150 minutes of
moderate-intensity exercise or 75 minutes
of vigorous-intensity exercise per week.

Protect Your Skin:
Protect your skin from the harmful effects
of ultraviolet (UV) radiation from the sun
and tanning beds. Use sunscreen with SPF
30 or higher, wear protective clothing,
seek shade during peak sun hours, and
avoid tanning beds.

Get Vaccinated:
Vaccines can help prevent certain cancer-causing infections. For example, the human papillomavirus (HPV) vaccine can protect against several HPV-related cancers, including cervical cancer.

Practice Safe Sex:
Practicing safe sex and reducing the number of sexual partners can lower the risk of sexually transmitted infections (STIs), such as HPV, which can lead to certain types of cancer.

Regular Screening and Health Checkups:
Regular cancer screenings and health checkups are essential for early detection and treatment of cancer. Follow recommended guidelines for screenings based on age, gender, and risk factors.

Manage Stress:
Chronic stress can impact overall health and may influence cancer risk indirectly. Adopting stress-reduction techniques,

such as mindfulness, meditation, or yoga, can help promote overall well-being. Remember that lifestyle modifications are most effective when combined. It's essential to create a comprehensive approach to health by incorporating multiple healthy habits. Additionally, it's important to consult with healthcare professionals for personalized guidance and to address any specific risk factors or concerns.

While lifestyle modifications can reduce the risk of cancer, it's crucial to remember that genetics and other factors also play a role in cancer development. Therefore, regular health checkups, screenings, and early detection remain vital components of cancer prevention and overall health management.

Vaccination and Cancer Prevention

Vaccination plays a critical role in cancer prevention by protecting against certain infections that are known to increase the risk of developing specific types of cancer. Some viruses and bacteria can cause chronic infections that lead to cellular changes and increase the likelihood of cancer development. Vaccines are designed to stimulate the immune system to recognize and fight these infectious agents, reducing the risk of associated cancers. Vaccination is an essential component of comprehensive cancer prevention strategies and has been proven to be highly effective in preventing certain cancer-related infections. Here are some key vaccinations that contribute to cancer prevention:

Human Papillomavirus (HPV) Vaccine: HPV is a common sexually transmitted infection that can cause several types of cancer, including cervical, vaginal, vulvar, penile, anal, and oropharyngeal cancers.

The HPV vaccine targets specific strains of the virus that are most strongly linked to cancer development.

The HPV vaccine is recommended for both males and females and is typically given in a series of two or three doses, depending on the age at which the vaccination begins.

Hepatitis B Vaccine:
Chronic infection with the hepatitis B virus (HBV) can lead to liver damage and increase the risk of liver cancer (hepatocellular carcinoma). The hepatitis B vaccine helps protect against HBV infection and its associated complications. The vaccine is usually given in a series of three or four doses.

Hepatitis C Treatment:
While there is no vaccine for hepatitis C (HCV), successful treatment and eradication of the virus in individuals with HCV infection can reduce the risk of liver cancer.

Vaccination not only benefits the vaccinated individuals but also contributes to population-wide immunity, known as herd immunity. When a significant portion of the population is vaccinated, it creates a protective barrier, making it difficult for infectious agents to spread. This indirectly protects those who are unvaccinated or unable to receive vaccines, such as individuals with weakened immune systems or certain medical conditions.

Vaccination is most effective when administered before exposure to the infectious agent, ideally during childhood or adolescence. However, catch-up vaccinations are also recommended for those who missed the recommended vaccination schedule.

It is essential to follow the vaccination guidelines provided by healthcare professionals and public health authorities. Routine health checkups and discussions with healthcare providers can help determine which vaccinations are appropriate for an individual based on age, medical history, and other factors.

Vaccination plays a crucial role in cancer prevention by protecting against certain infections known to increase the risk of specific cancers. The HPV vaccine and hepatitis B vaccine have been particularly effective in reducing the incidence of associated cancers. By preventing cancer-related infections through vaccination, we can make significant strides in reducing the burden of preventable cancers and improving public health.

Promising research and the road ahead in cancer treatment hold the potential for significant advancements in the fight against cancer. Over the years, groundbreaking discoveries and innovative technologies have led to improved outcomes for cancer patients. As the field of oncology continues to evolve, researchers and healthcare professionals are focused on various areas of investigation to further enhance cancer prevention, early detection, diagnosis, and treatment. Here are some key areas of promising research and developments in cancer treatment:

Immunotherapy Advancements: Immunotherapy has revolutionized cancer treatment by harnessing the body's immune system to recognize and attack cancer cells. Immune checkpoint inhibitors, CAR T-cell therapy, and other

immunotherapies have shown remarkable success in treating certain types of cancer, including melanoma, lung cancer, and hematological malignancies.
Ongoing research aims to expand the applications of immunotherapy to other cancer types, improve response rates, and overcome resistance to treatment.
Precision Medicine and Personalized

Therapy:
Precision oncology involves tailoring cancer treatment to an individual's specific genetic profile, allowing for more targeted and effective therapies. Advances in genomic sequencing and molecular profiling have enabled researchers to identify specific genetic alterations driving cancer growth.
Precision medicine allows oncologists to match patients with targeted therapies or clinical trials based on their tumor's unique characteristics, increasing the likelihood of treatment success.

Gene Editing and Gene Therapies:
Gene editing technologies like CRISPR-Cas9 hold promise in modifying cancer cells to improve the body's ability to fight cancer. Researchers are exploring gene editing approaches to disable oncogenes, enhance tumor suppressors, or make cancer cells more susceptible to treatments. Gene therapies, such as CAR T-cell therapy, continue to be refined and expanded to target a broader range of cancer types and improve safety and efficacy.

Targeting Cancer Stem Cells:
Cancer stem cells are a small subset of cells within tumors that are believed to drive cancer growth and recurrence. Targeting these cells could lead to more durable and long-lasting responses to treatment.
Research is ongoing to identify effective therapies that specifically target cancer stem cells and disrupt their ability to sustain tumor growth.

Nanotechnology and Drug Delivery:
Nanotechnology offers exciting opportunities in cancer treatment by improving drug delivery systems. Nanoparticles can carry therapeutic agents directly to tumor sites, enhancing drug effectiveness while reducing toxicity to healthy tissues.
Researchers are exploring various nanoparticle formulations and delivery methods to optimize treatment outcomes.

Liquid Biopsies and Early Detection:
Liquid biopsies, which involve analyzing blood or other body fluids for cancer-specific biomarkers, are being developed as a non-invasive method for early cancer detection and monitoring treatment response.
Early detection is crucial in improving cancer outcomes, and liquid biopsies may play a significant role in diagnosing cancer at earlier stages.

Artificial Intelligence and Machine Learning:
AI and machine learning algorithms have the potential to analyze vast amounts of medical data and assist in diagnosis, treatment planning, and predicting treatment outcomes.
These technologies may aid in identifying patterns and potential therapeutic targets, guiding personalized treatment decisions for individual patients.
Despite these promising advancements, challenges remain in cancer research and treatment. Ensuring the accessibility and affordability of new therapies, overcoming drug resistance, and addressing potential long-term side effects are areas of ongoing investigation.

Promising research and advancements in cancer treatment offer hope for improved outcomes and quality of life for cancer patients. Collaborations between researchers, healthcare providers, and pharmaceutical companies are essential to furthering scientific discoveries and translating them into effective treatments. As technology and knowledge continue to advance, the future of cancer treatment holds the promise of more targeted, personalized, and effective therapies, ultimately leading to better cancer outcomes and improved patient care.

Conclusion

Cancer is a complex and multifaceted disease that continues to challenge the medical community and impact millions of lives worldwide. Throughout this comprehensive exploration of cancer-related topics, we have delved into the fundamental aspects of cancer, including its definition, causes, development, diagnosis, staging, and treatment options. We have also explored the crucial role of lifestyle modifications and vaccination in cancer prevention, as well as the importance of psychological and emotional support for patients and their families.

Understanding cancer involves recognizing its diverse origins, ranging from genetic factors to environmental exposures, and the intricate cellular processes that drive tumorigenesis and metastasis. Accurate cancer diagnosis, staging, and grading are essential for devising appropriate treatment plans that may encompass conventional therapies, targeted therapies, and emerging experimental approaches like gene therapy and nanotechnology.

Beyond treatment, supporting patients throughout their cancer journey is equally vital. Effective symptom management, palliative care, and end-of-life care provide comfort, dignity, and support to patients and their families during challenging times.

Encouraging research and promising advancements in cancer treatment, such as immunotherapy, precision medicine, gene editing, and nanotechnology, fuel hope for more effective and targeted therapies in the future. Collaborations between researchers, healthcare providers, and advocacy groups contribute to a deeper understanding of cancer biology and treatment strategies, paving the way for better patient outcomes and quality of life.

Prevention remains a cornerstone in the battle against cancer, and lifestyle modifications, vaccination, and early detection play significant roles in reducing cancer risk and improving overall public health.

As the field of oncology evolves, there is an ongoing commitment to fostering progress and innovation to ultimately achieve the goal of eradicating cancer. While challenges persist, the collective efforts of the medical community, patients, caregivers, and society as a whole will continue to drive advancements in cancer research, treatment, and supportive care. Above all, at the heart of this exploration is the unwavering dedication to cancer patients, survivors, and their families. Through education, compassionate care, and ongoing research, we strive to improve cancer outcomes, alleviate suffering, and provide hope for a future where cancer is more effectively prevented, diagnosed, and treated.

Together, we stand united in the fight against cancer, determined to create a world where the burden of this devastating disease is reduced, and where all individuals have the opportunity to live healthy and fulfilling lives.